This Journal Belongs to:

_____

If lost, please contact:

_____

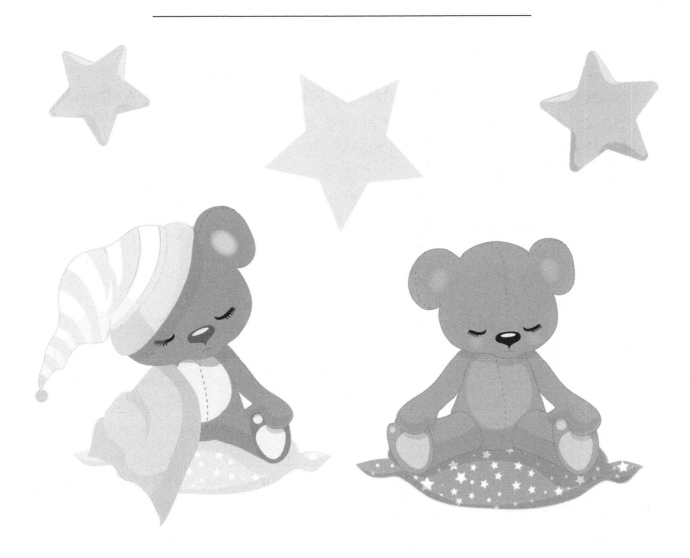

Here's what you can expect in this Pregnancy journal:

This is such an exciting time in your lives! **This journal assumes two daddies have a surrogate who is pregnant with your beautiful baby.** Be sure to scan the whole journal right away so you know where to find everything described below, so that you can get the most out of it.

- "Our Journey of Surrogacy" journaling pages
- "We Are Pregnant" Journal Page to record details of when you first found out you were going to be daddies.
- "Our Pregnancy Journal" Pages - Weeks 4 – 41 – to record our weekly memories of the pregnancy, plus extra space for free thought journaling (**Hint:** Use the Journal Prompt Ideas included)
- 3 journal pages to summarize each of the trimesters
- Space for both dads to write "My First Love Letter to My Baby"
- Space for listing your Baby Name Ideas
- Newborn Baby Shopping List
- Hospital Bag Checklist
- Our Baby Shower
- Our Sonogram Photos
- Our Birth Plan
- Our Nursery Room Ideas
- Our Family Tree (includes both Daddies)
- Important Pre-Birth Questions & Considerations
- The Birth Day

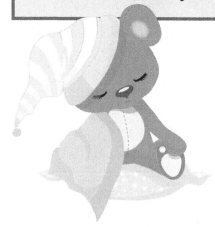

Our Journey of Surrogacy

How long it took to find our surrogate, how we found her, why we chose her, her age, history, etc.

_____

_____

_____

_____

_____

_____

_____

_____

_____

_____

_____

_____

_____

_____

_____

_____

_____

_____

_____

_____

_____

_____

_____

_____

_____

_____

Our Journey of Surrogacy

We Are Pregnant!

Date we found out: _____

How far along was the pregnancy?: _____

How we found out: _____

Our Estimated Due Date:

_____

_____

_____

_____

Our reactions: _____

_____

_____

_____

Did we suspect we were pregnant?: _____

_____

_____

_____

Who we first told about the pregnancy & their reactions: _____

_____

_____

_____

What else do we remember about the day we found out that we were expecting our baby?:

_____

_____

_____

_____

_____

_____

_____

Journal Prompts & Ideas to Write About

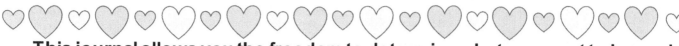

This journal allows you the freedom to determine what you want to journal about on each page that represents a different week of the pregnancy.

Here are some ideas to get your creative juices flowing:
- How the two of you met
- Where you were both born
- Where the two of you went to school, college, etc.
- What kinds of jobs you have had
- What you are now doing to earn money for a living
- Why and when you decided you wanted a baby
- The process of finding your surrogate
- Who your siblings and families are
- What you are most looking forward to about becoming fathers
- What your hopes and dreams are for your baby
- What is the most difficult time you have ever had in your life, and how did you get through it?
- What have hard times in life taught you that are important for your child to know?
- What do you want your baby to know about you?
- Is there anything about your life that you would go back and change, and why?
- Who are the grandparents and what is their history (birth dates, where grew up, went to school, their siblings, etc.)?

List more of your ideas, that you don't want to forget, to write about in this journal:

_____

_____

_____

_____

_____

_____

_____

Our Pregnancy Journal 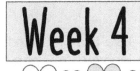 Week 4

What we want to remember most about this week:

_____
_____
_____
_____
_____
_____
_____
_____
_____

Photo of Your Daddies Before You Were Born:

Date:

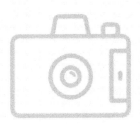

Use this page and subsequent ones to write freely about your life stories and the pregnancy journey. You can also use this space to paste photos that you want to share with your baby.

Our Pregnancy Journal

What we want to remember most about this week:

Another photo of your Daddies

Date:

Our baby's tissues & organ systems begin to develop in Week 5.

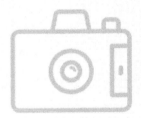

Our Pregnancy Journal

What we want to remember most about this week:

The neural tube in baby's back closes, heart & other organs are developing, small arm buds appear, & eyes & ears primitively form.

Insert your own topic you want to share with your unborn baby here & on subsequent pages (use Journal Prompt ideas near the front of this journal).

Date:

Our Pregnancy Journal

What we want to remember most about this week:

Baby's brain & head are growing, nostrils and retinas are starting to develop, leg buds appear, & the arm buds look like paddles.

Date:

Baby has doubled in size since last week, and is now the size of a blueberry.

Our Pregnancy Journal

Week 8

♡♡♡♡♡♡♡♡♡♡♡♡♡♡♡♡

What we want to remember most about this week:

Fingers and nose are forming, and the leg buds look like paddles.

Date:

Baby is the size of a kidney bean, and over ½" long.

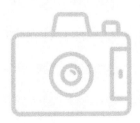

A picture of our home before you were born

Our Pregnancy Journal

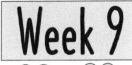

Week 9

What we want to remember most about this week:

Baby's eyelids form, baby's arms grow, elbows appear, & toes are developing.

Date:

Baby is the size of a grape. The eyes are fully formed, but closed.

Our Pregnancy Journal
Week 10

What we want to remember most about this week:

_____
_____
_____
_____
_____
_____
_____
_____
_____

Baby can bend the elbows, the toes & fingers aren't as webbed in appearance as they get longer, and the head gets rounder.

Date:

Baby is the size of a kumquat, measures a bit over 1" from head to buttocks.

_____
_____
_____
_____
_____
_____
_____
_____
_____
_____
_____
_____

Our Pregnancy Journal   Week 11

What we want to remember most about this week:

Baby is inhaling & exhaling small amounts of amniotic fluid, exercising the lungs.

Date:

Baby is the size of a fig, over 1.5" long, & can kick & stretch..

Our Pregnancy Journal

What we want to remember most about this week:

Baby's muscles are getting bigger, & baby is opening & closing his/her fingers, and kicking his/her arms and legs.

Date:

Baby is the size of a lime, and is over 2" long from head to baby's butt.

Our First Trimester

What we enjoyed most about the first trimester

How We Felt This Trimester

Our Favorite Memories

Our Pregnancy Journal

What we want to remember most about this week:

Baby's body is catching up to the growth of his head. All essential organs & body systems have developed, baby's kidneys are working, testicles or ovaries are formed, fingerprints are starting.

Date:

Baby is the size of a pea pod, approx. 3" long, & weighs 1 oz.

Our Pregnancy Journal

What we want to remember most about this week:

Baby exhibits sucking reflexes, and is growing fine-like hair (lanugo) to help regulate his/her temperature.

Date:

Baby is the size of a lemon, 3.5" long, & can make some facial expressions.

Our Pregnancy Journal

What we want to remember most about this week:

Baby's bones are hardening, muscles continue to form, &
baby's closed eyes are starting to be sensitive to light.

Date:

Baby is the size of an apple, 4" long, &
2.5 oz..

Our Pregnancy Journal

What we want to remember most about this week:

Baby's heart is pumping around 49 pints (28 L) of blood around his/her body every day!

Date:

Baby is the size of an avocado, 4.5 long, 3.5 oz.

Our Pregnancy Journal

What we want to remember most about this week:

Baby's hearing is pretty good, & can hear your muffled voice & music. Your baby has his own set of distinct fingerprints.

Date:

Baby is the size of a turnip, weighs 5 oz, & is 5" long..

Our Pregnancy Journal

What we want to remember most about this week:

Post a picture of something Daddy enjoys doing.

Date:

Baby is the size of a bell pepper, weighs 7 oz. & is 5.5 long..
Baby is growing eyebrows.

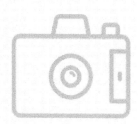

Our Pregnancy Journal

What we want to remember most about this week:

Hair may be beginning to grow on baby's head, the brain is specializing, & the surrogate may be feeling baby's movements at this point.

Date:

Baby is the size of a large tomato, weighs 8.5 oz. & is 6" long.

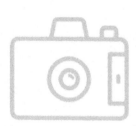

Here's a picture of my other Daddy doing something he enjoys.

Our Pregnancy Journal

What we want to remember most about this week:

The pregnancy is halfway done! Baby is moving a lot within the womb now.

Date:

Baby is the size of a banana, & is 6.5" from head to butt or 10" to the heels.

Our Pregnancy Journal

What we want to remember most about this week:

If you are feeling baby's movements, you will begin to recognize periods of wakefulness and sleeping. Baby's eyes move rapidly under the eyelids.

Date:

Baby is 10.5" long (like a carrot, & weighs approximately 12 oz.

Our Pregnancy Journal

What we want to remember most about this week:

Baby's fingernails are clearly visible. Meconium (which will be baby's first poop) is developing in the bowels.

Date:

Baby is the size of a spaghetti squash, weighs 1 lb, & is 11" long from head to butt.

Our Pregnancy Journal

What we want to remember most about this week:

Baby's hearing is improving to hear other sounds outside of the womb.

Date:

Baby is the size of a large mango.

Our Pregnancy Journal
Week 24

What we want to remember most about this week:

_____
_____
_____
_____
_____
_____
_____
_____
_____
_____
_____

Baby is considered possibly "viable" if he/she is born now, but really needs more time to grow & maximize the chances for survival outside the womb. Your baby makes facial expressions.

Date:

Baby is about 12" (30 cm) long, & weighs 1 ¼ lb.

_____
_____
_____
_____
_____
_____
_____
_____
_____
_____
_____

Our Pregnancy Journal   Week 25

What we want to remember most about this week:

Here's a photo of _____

Date:

Baby is the size of a rutabaga. It is about 13.5" in length, & 1 ½ lb.
Baby is putting on more fat in preparation for birth.

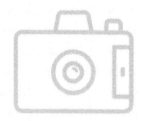

Our Pregnancy Journal

What we want to remember most about this week:

Baby can recognize voices. Baby's tastebuds are developed. The lungs continue to develop.

Date:

Baby is 14" long, 1 & 2/3 lb.

Our Pregnancy Journal

What we want to remember most about this week:

The surrogate may feel when your baby hiccups. Baby is also experiencing more regular patterns of sleep and wakefulness, which the surrogate may start to notice.

Date:

Baby is the size of a cauliflower, is 14.5 long, & 2 lb in weight.

Our Pregnancy Journal   Week 28

What we want to remember most about this week:

Baby's eyes now open & close, have eyelashes, & can form tears. The irises are now pigmented.

Date:

Baby is the size of an eggplant, weighs 2 ¼ lb., & is 15" long.

Our Second Trimester

Weeks 13-28

What we enjoyed most & least about the second trimester

_____
_____
_____
_____
_____
_____
_____
_____
_____

How We Felt This Trimester

_____
_____
_____
_____
_____
_____

Our Favorite Memories

_____
_____
_____
_____
_____
_____
_____
_____

Our Pregnancy Journal
Week 29

What we want to remember most about this week:

Baby's brain continues to develop the neurons needed for intelligence & personality.

Date:

Baby is the size of a butternut squash, 15" long, & 2.5 lb.

Our Pregnancy Journal

What we want to remember most about this week:

When a flashlight is shone on the belly, you may notice your baby move or kick.

Date:

Baby is the size of a big cabbage, weighs 3 lb. & is 15 ¾" long.

Our Pregnancy Journal
Week 31

What we want to remember most about this week:

Baby is getting longer & bigger, so he/she takes on the curled-up, fetal position in utero until birth now.

Date:

Baby is the weight of a coconut.

Our Pregnancy Journal
Week 32

What we want to remember most about this week:

If born now, baby has a good chance of surviving & being healthy, although baby's lungs aren't fully developed yet.

Date:

Baby is 16 ¾" long, & weighs approx. 3 ¾ lb..

Our Pregnancy Journal
Week 33

What we want to remember most about this week:

You may notice that your baby's activity level & responses are dependent on your own actions, such as whether you've just eaten or you're in a noisy environment.

Date:

Baby is the weight of a pineapple, weighs 4 lb, & is 17" long..

Our Pregnancy Journal Week 34

What we want to remember most about this week:

This is a great time to sing lullabies to your baby, as baby is more likely to recognize them after birth.

Date:

Baby is 18" long, & 4 ¾ lb.

Our Pregnancy Journal
Week 35

What we want to remember most about this week:

The amniotic fluid surrounding baby is decreasing. 97% of babies are head-down at this point, in preparation for the birth.

Date:

Baby is the weight of a large honeydew melon at 5 ¼ lb..

Our Pregnancy Journal

Week 36

What we want to remember most about this week:

Baby is shedding the lanugo hair & vernix caseosa (white waxy substance) this week. Baby's sucking is fully developed now.

Date:

Baby is 18.5" long, & weighs close to 6 lb.

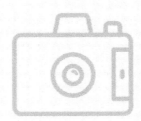

This is a photo of our excited faces as we wait for your arrival!

Our Pregnancy Journal Week 37

What we want to remember most about this week:

Your surrogate passes antibodies to your baby through the umbilical cord. Baby's grasp is improving, ready to grasp your fingers (and hearts) when born.

Date:

Baby is approximately 19" long, & 6 1/3 lb.

Our Pregnancy Journal   Week 38

What we want to remember most about this week:

Baby continues to improve his/her breathing, circulation, & digestion.

Date:

Baby weighs about 7 lb. & is 19.5" long.

Our Pregnancy Journal   Week 39

What we want to remember most about this week:

If you haven't met baby yet, baby is ready to meet his/her daddies any day now!

Date:

Baby is the weight of a watermelon, around 7 lb.

Our Pregnancy Journal
Week 40

What we want to remember most about this week:

Your baby will be born with many natural reflexes necessary for survival (rooting for the nipple, suckling, etc.)

Date:

Baby is the size of a pumpkin, weighs approx. 7.5 lb. & 20" long.

Our Pregnancy Journal
Week 41

What we want to remember most about this week:

It should be any time now! Have you decided on a name yet?

Date:

Our Third Trimester

What we enjoyed most & least about the third trimester

_____
_____
_____
_____
_____
_____
_____
_____

How We Felt This Trimester

_____
_____
_____
_____
_____
_____

Our Favorite Memories

_____
_____
_____
_____
_____
_____

Our Baby Name Ideas

Girl's Names

Boy's Names

Other thoughts:

My First Love Letter to My Unborn Baby

My First Love Letter to My Unborn Baby

_____
_____
_____
_____
_____
_____
_____
_____
_____
_____
_____
_____
_____
_____
_____
_____
_____
_____
_____
_____
_____
_____
_____
_____
_____
_____
_____
_____
_____

Nursery Room Ideas

Favorite website examples: _____

_____

_____

_____

_____

_____

_____

Color scheme & theme ideas: _____

_____

_____

_____

_____

_____

_____

Draw out the layout, or add more notes:

Our Baby Shower

Friends & family who attended:

Games we played:

Baby Shower Photo:

Our Favorite Memories of the Day:

More memorable details of our shower, including gifts received, or photos, etc.

Our Sonogram Photos

We loved you before you were born, little one.

Newborn Baby Shopping Checklist

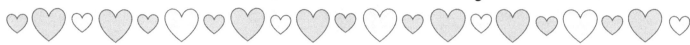

TIP: Keep in mind that baby grows quickly so don't buy too many clothes or diapers of the same size before baby is born. Don't forget to sign up for prenatal classes and Baby CPR classes.

Clothing

- [ ] Onesies
- [ ] Sleepwear
- [ ] Undershirts
- [ ] Socks
- [ ] Slippers
- [ ] Pants or shorts
- [ ] Shirts
- [ ] Dresses
- [ ] Scratch prevention mittens
- [ ] Baby hat
- [ ] Sweaters and jackets for babies born in cool weather
- [ ] Snowsuit & mitts for baby born in winter

Sleeping

- [ ] Crib & mattress
- [ ] Sheets for crib
- [ ] Baby monitor
- [ ] Swaddling blankets
- [ ] Baby sling
- [ ]
- [ ]

Bathing

- [ ] Baby wash cloths
- [ ] Baby hooded towels
- [ ] Soft-bristled baby brush
- [ ] Baby body wash/shampoo
- [ ] Baby lotion
- [ ] Baby bathtub
- [ ]
- [ ]
- [ ]

Diapering

- [ ] Diaper rash ointment
- [ ] Diaper pad &/or change table
- [ ] Baby wipes
- [ ] Diapers
- [ ] Diaper pail
- [ ] Diaper bag
- [ ]
- [ ]
- [ ]

Feeding

- [ ] Formula
- [ ] Baby bottles, bottle liners, bottle brush
- [ ] Burp cloths & receiving blankets
- [ ] Bibs
- [ ] High chair
- [ ]
- [ ]
- [ ]
- [ ]

Miscellaneous

- [ ] Baby laundry detergent
- [ ] Infant car seat
- [ ] Stroller
- [ ] Baby thermometer
- [ ] Mobile for crib
- [ ] Rocking chair
- [ ] Night light
- [ ] Nasal bulb syringe
- [ ] Nail scissors
- [ ] Pacifiers
- [ ] Baby swing

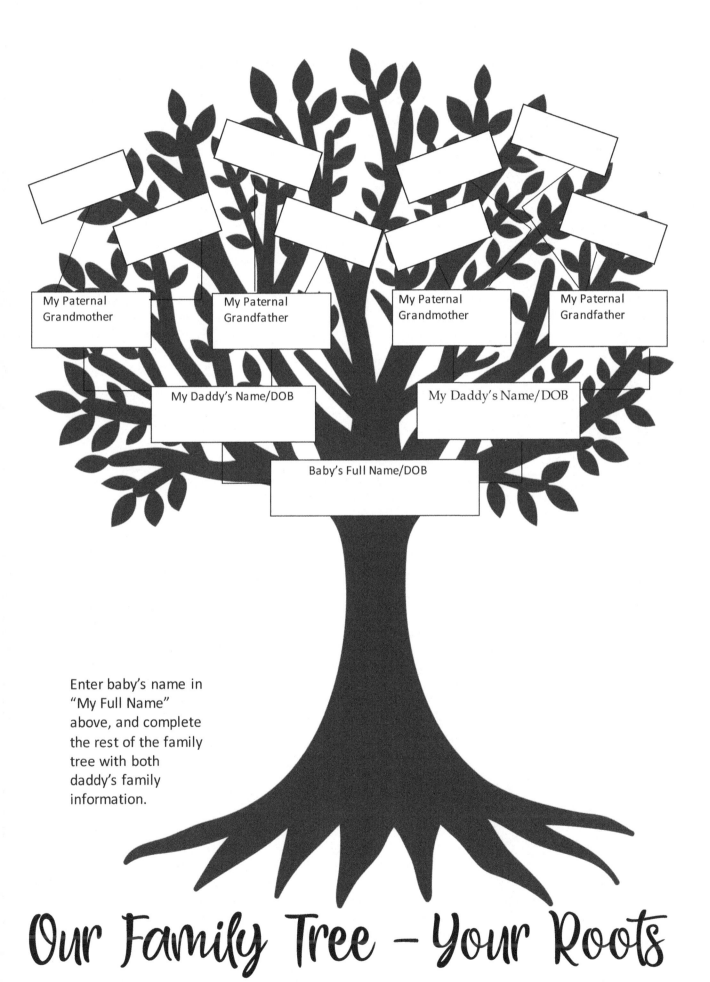

My Paternal Grandmother

My Paternal Grandfather

My Paternal Grandmother

My Paternal Grandfather

My Daddy's Name/DOB

My Daddy's Name/DOB

Baby's Full Name/DOB

Enter baby's name in "My Full Name" above, and complete the rest of the family tree with both daddy's family information.

Our Family Tree – Your Roots

Create your own family tree from scratch if you need to represent divorces or deaths, and
resulting remarriages that may have occurred in your families.

Baby's full name/DOB

Important Pre-Birth Questions

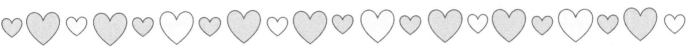

Do we want a midwife or obstetrician caring for our surrogate during the pregnancy, and why are we choosing one over the other?

What values are important to us when choosing our midwife or obstetrician (i.e. belief in natural process, etc.)?

Is cord blood banking something we want to consider, and if so, where can we learn more?

If we have a boy, what are our thoughts on circumcision, and the risks and benefits?

Post more of our questions below:

Our Birth Plan

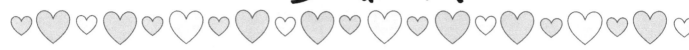

Who we want present at the birth: _____
_____
_____

Surrogate's preferences for pain control: _____
_____
_____
_____

Our agreed preferences re: medical interventions during labor: _____
_____
_____

Our agreed preferences for medical interventions during _____
delivery: _____
_____
_____
_____

Who will cut the umbilical cord: _____

How we plan to feed our baby after birth: _____
_____

Most important issues to us: _____
_____
_____
_____

Other: _____
_____
_____
_____
_____

Hospital Bag Checklist

⭐ For Both Daddies ⭐

- [ ] Medical cards & insurance documents
- [ ] Birth plan
- [ ] Lip balm
- [ ] Snacks & water
- [ ] Deodorant/antiperspirant
- [ ] Change of clothes
- [ ] Phone, camera, video camera, & chargers
- [ ] Glasses, contacts, solution
- [ ] Money/credit card
- [ ] Hair brush
- [ ] Book
- [ ] Toothbrush, toothpaste, & floss
- [ ]
- [ ]
- [ ]
- [ ]
- [ ]
- [ ]
- [ ]
- [ ]
- [ ]

- [ ]
- [ ]
- [ ]
- [ ]
- [ ]
- [ ]
- [ ]
- [ ]
- [ ]
- [ ]
- [ ]
- [ ]

⭐ For Baby

- [ ] Nightgown
- [ ] Sleepers
- [ ] Car seat
- [ ] Going-home outfit
- [ ] Socks & slippers
- [ ] Outerwear appropriate for the season
- [ ] Receiving blankets
- [ ] Pacifier
- [ ] Bottle & formula
- [ ]
- [ ]
- [ ]
- [ ]

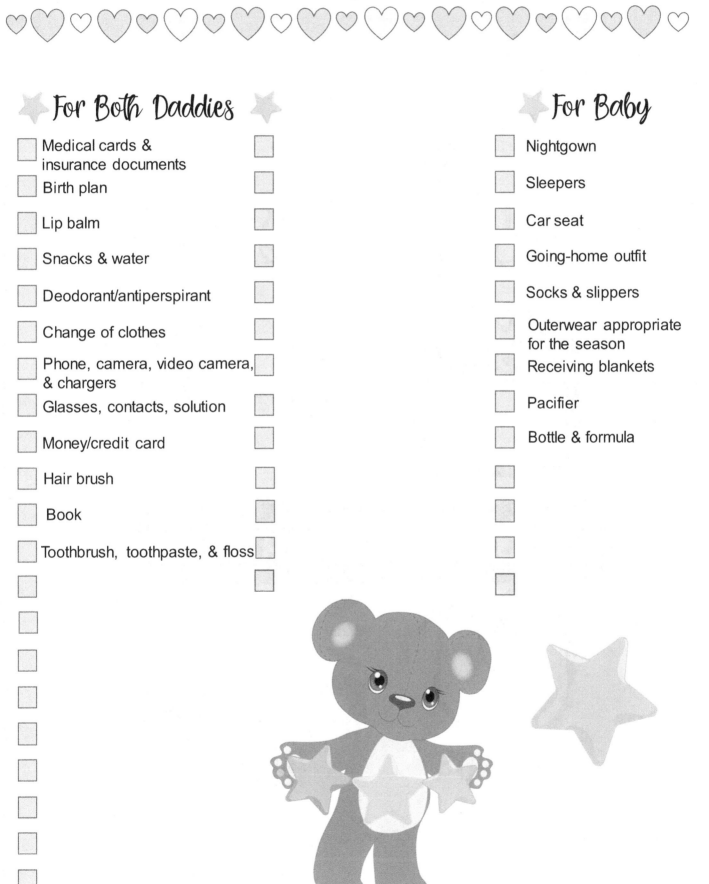

The Birth

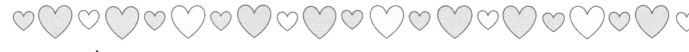

Baby's Full Name: _____

WELCOME TO THE WORLD!

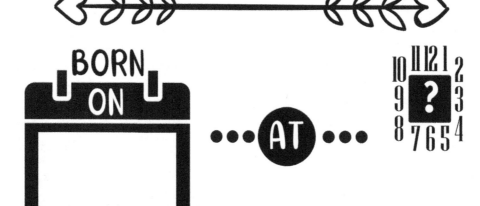

BORN ON

···· AT ····

WEIGHING & MEASURING

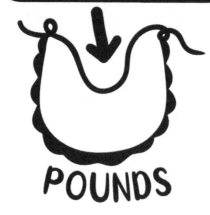

POUNDS

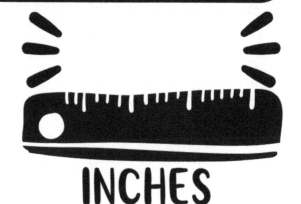

INCHES

First photo of our baby

More photos of baby and Daddies

Made in United States
Orlando, FL
01 April 2022

16384641R00057